This Book

Belongs to:

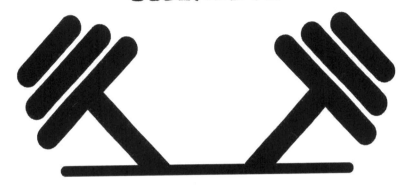

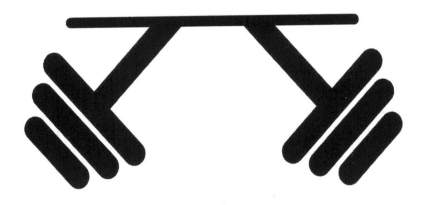

WHAT IS MY WHY?

Take a minute to write down some powerful thoughts. What's your real "Why"? What is your biggest motivation? This is the page you'll come back to when you feel tiered and not committed to the challenge. This will be a reminder of why you are taking this 75 day challenge and why you are trying to take care of your body and your health.

FITNESS GOAL

START DATE :

DURATION :

END DATE :

START WEIGHT :

GOAL WEIGHT :

FINAL BMI :

START BMI :

GOAL BMI :

FINAL WEIGHT :

HABIT

NEW HABITS TO BUILD

BAD HABITS TO CUT

MEASUREMENTS		
	START	END
BUST		
WAIST		
HIPS		
CHEST		
THIGHS		
ARM		

MOTIVATION/BIG WHY

NOTES

Year
PLAN

YEAR:

January

_____
_____
_____
_____
_____

February

_____
_____
_____
_____
_____

March

_____
_____
_____
_____
_____

April

_____
_____
_____
_____
_____

May

_____
_____
_____
_____
_____

June

_____
_____
_____
_____
_____

July

_____
_____
_____
_____
_____

August

_____
_____
_____
_____
_____

September

_____
_____
_____
_____
_____

October

_____
_____
_____
_____
_____

November

_____
_____
_____
_____
_____

December

_____
_____
_____
_____
_____

My Weight Loss Journey

	Starting Weight	Ending Weight	+/- Pounds
Week 1			
Week 2			
Week 3			
Week 4			
Week 5			
Week 6			
Week 7			
Week 8			
Week 9			
Week 10			

WEIGHT TRACKER

MONTH: YEAR:

DATE	WEIGHT	GAIN+	LOSS+	NOTES

WEIGHT TRACKER

MONTH: YEAR:

DATE	WEIGHT	GAIN+	LOSS+	NOTES

WEIGHT TRACKER

MONTH: YEAR:

DATE	WEIGHT	GAIN+	LOSS+	NOTES

WEIGHT TRACKER

MONTH:				YEAR:

DATE	WEIGHT	GAIN+	LOSS+	NOTES

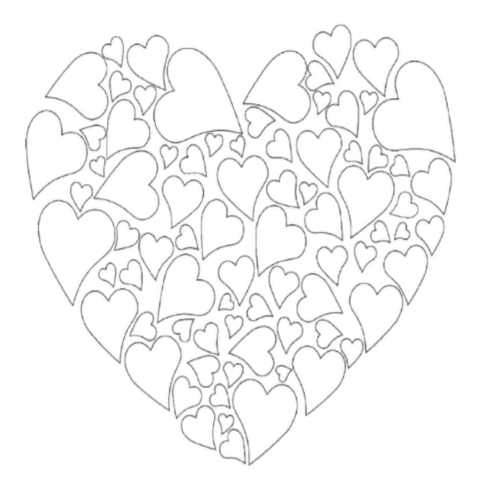

-》》》》 COLOR YOUR DAY 《《《《-

RED

If Completed

Yellow

If Completed
partially
(e.g. missed out fitness log,
water intake etc.)

Black

If Skipped

Monthly
PLAN

MONTH:

SUNDAY					
MONDAY					
TUESDAY					
WEDNESDAY					
THURSDAY					
FRIDAY					
SATURDAY					

WEEKLY MEAL GOAL

MONTH OF :

	BREAKFAST	LUNCH	DINNER	SNACKS	NOTES
MONDAY					
TUESDAY					
WEDNESDAY					
THURSDAY					
FRIDAY					
SATURDAY					
SUNDAY					

Fitness Workout Planner

Date: Year: Month:

	Activity	Reps
Day 1		
Day 2		
Day 3		
Day 4		
Day 5		
Day 6		
Day 7		

Weekly

PLAN

WEEK:

SUNDAY	
MONDAY	
TUESDAY	
WEDNESDAY	
THURSDAY	
FRIDAY	
SATURDAY	

To do

-
-
-
-
-
-
-
-

Tracker

S M T W T F S

S M T W T F S

S M T W T F S

Notes

MY JOURNAL

WEEKLY REVIEW

Date: ....

Week: 1 2 3 4

HOW WAS THE WEEK?

FELT GRATEFUL THIS WEEK FOR:

THIS WEEK'S SMALL WINS

THINGS I HAVE IMPROVED ON:

TASK IN PROGRESS

THIS WEEK'S BAD EXPERIENCE:

WHAT TO NOTE THIS WEEK:

MY JOURNAL

WEEKLY WRITING

Date: _____

Week: 1   2   3   4

dream,
believe,
achieve

WEEKLY MEAL GOAL

MONTH OF :

	BREAKFAST	LUNCH	DINNER	SNACKS	NOTES
MONDAY					
TUESDAY					
WEDNESDAY					
THURSDAY					
FRIDAY					
SATURDAY					
SUNDAY					

Fitness Workout Planner

Date: Year: Month:

	Activity	Reps
Day 1		
Day 2		
Day 3		
Day 4		
Day 5		
Day 6		
Day 7		

Weekly
PLAN

WEEK:

SUNDAY	
MONDAY	
TUESDAY	
WEDNESDAY	
THURSDAY	
FRIDAY	
SATURDAY	

To do

-
-
-
-
-
-
-
-

Tracker

S M T W T F S

S M T W T F S

S M T W T F S

Notes

MY JOURNAL

WEEKLY REVIEW

Date: ....

Week: 1 2 3 4

HOW WAS THE WEEK?

FELT GRATEFUL THIS WEEK FOR:

THIS WEEK'S SMALL WINS

THINGS I HAVE IMPROVED ON:

TASK IN PROGRESS

THIS WEEK'S BAD EXPERIENCE:

WHAT TO NOTE THIS WEEK:

MY JOURNAL

WEEKLY WRITING

Date: _____

Week: 1 2 3 4

HELLO JOURNAL, MY WEEK IS…

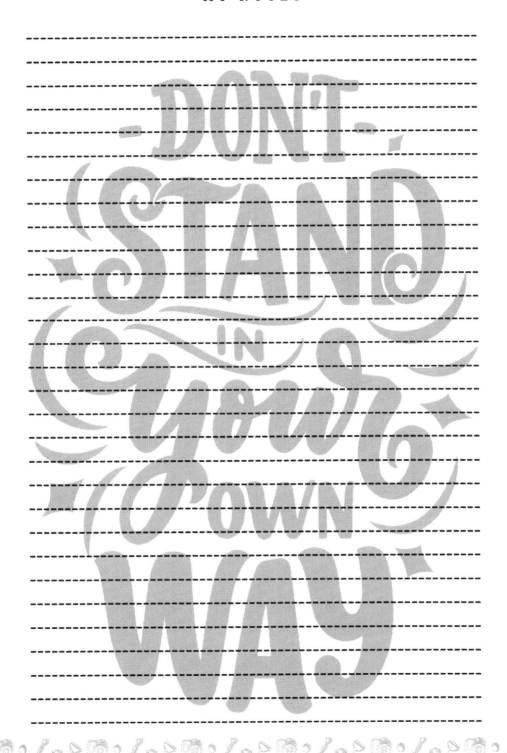

WEEKLY MEAL GOAL

MONTH OF :

	BREAKFAST	LUNCH	DINNER	SNACKS	NOTES
MONDAY					
TUESDAY					
WEDNESDAY					
THURSDAY					
FRIDAY					
SATURDAY					
SUNDAY					

Fitness Workout Planner

Date: Year: Month:

	Activity	Reps
Day 1		
Day 2		
Day 3		
Day 4		
Day 5		
Day 6		
Day 7		

Weekly
PLAN

WEEK:

SUNDAY

MONDAY

TUESDAY

WEDNESDAY

THURSDAY

FRIDAY

SATURDAY

To do

Tracker

S M T W T F S

S M T W T F S

S M T W T F S

Notes

MY JOURNAL

WEEKLY REVIEW

Date: ....

Week: 1 2 3 4

HOW WAS THE WEEK?

FELT GRATEFUL THIS WEEK FOR:

THIS WEEK'S SMALL WINS

THINGS I HAVE IMPROVED ON:

TASK IN PROGRESS

THIS WEEK'S BAD EXPERIENCE:

WHAT TO NOTE THIS WEEK:

MY JOURNAL

WEEKLY WRITING

Date: ....

Week: 1 2 3 4

HELLO JOURNAL, MY WEEK IS...

EVERY JOURNEY NEEDS A FIRST STEP

WEEKLY MEAL GOAL

MONTH OF :

	BREAKFAST	LUNCH	DINNER	SNACKS	NOTES
MONDAY					
TUESDAY					
WEDNESDAY					
THURSDAY					
FRIDAY					
SATURDAY					
SUNDAY					

Fitness Workout Planner

Date: Year: Month:

	Activity	Reps
Day 1		
Day 2		
Day 3		
Day 4		
Day 5		
Day 6		
Day 7		

Weekly

PLAN

WEEK:

SUNDAY

MONDAY

TUESDAY

WEDNESDAY

THURSDAY

FRIDAY

SATURDAY

To do

- [ ] _____
- [ ] _____
- [ ] _____
- [ ] _____
- [ ] _____
- [ ] _____
- [ ] _____
- [ ] _____

Tracker

S	M	T	W	T	F	S

S	M	T	W	T	F	S

S	M	T	W	T	F	S

Notes

MY JOURNAL

WEEKLY REVIEW

Date: _____

Week: 1 2 3 4

HOW WAS THE WEEK?

FELT GRATEFUL THIS WEEK FOR:

THIS WEEK'S SMALL WINS

THINGS I HAVE IMPROVED ON:

TASK IN PROGRESS

THIS WEEK'S BAD EXPERIENCE:

WHAT TO NOTE THIS WEEK:

MY JOURNAL

WEEKLY WRITING

Date: _____

Week: 1 2 3 4

HELLO JOURNAL, MY WEEK IS...

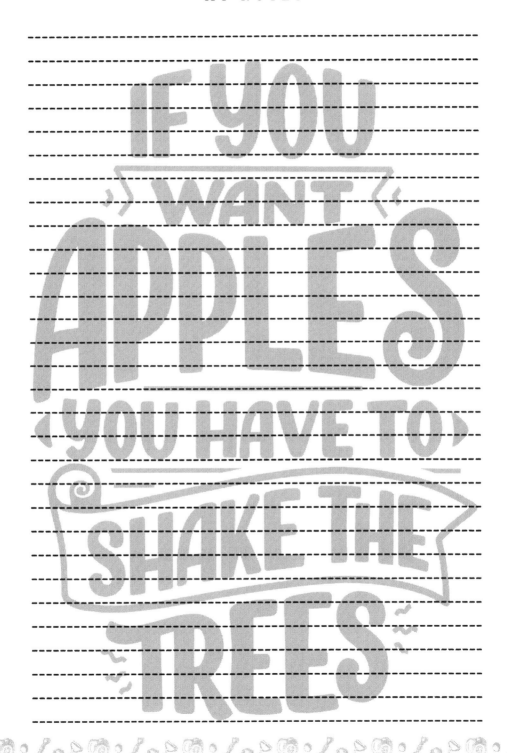

Monthly
PLAN

SUNDAY					
MONDAY					
TUESDAY					
WEDNESDAY					
THURSDAY					
FRIDAY					
SATURDAY					

WEEKLY MEAL GOAL

MONTH OF :

	BREAKFAST	LUNCH	DINNER	SNACKS	NOTES
MONDAY					
TUESDAY					
WEDNESDAY					
THURSDAY					
FRIDAY					
SATURDAY					
SUNDAY					

Fitness Workout Planner

Date: Year: Month:

	Activity	Reps
Day 1		
Day 2		
Day 3		
Day 4		
Day 5		
Day 6		
Day 7		

Weekly
PLAN

WEEK:

SUNDAY	
MONDAY	
TUESDAY	
WEDNESDAY	
THURSDAY	
FRIDAY	
SATURDAY	

To do

- ☐ ....
- ☐ ....
- ☐ ....
- ☐ ....
- ☐ ....
- ☐ ....
- ☐ ....
- ☐ ....

Tracker

S	M	T	W	T	F	S
☐	☐	☐	☐	☐	☐	☐

S	M	T	W	T	F	S
☐	☐	☐	☐	☐	☐	☐

S	M	T	W	T	F	S
☐	☐	☐	☐	☐	☐	☐

Notes

MY JOURNAL

WEEKLY REVIEW

HOW WAS THE WEEK?

FELT GRATEFUL THIS WEEK FOR:

THIS WEEK'S SMALL WINS

THINGS I HAVE IMPROVED ON:

TASK IN PROGRESS

THIS WEEK'S BAD EXPERIENCE:

WHAT TO NOTE THIS WEEK:

MY JOURNAL

WEEKLY WRITING

Date: ....

Week: 1   2   3   4

HELLO JOURNAL, MY WEEK IS...

WEEKLY MEAL GOAL

MONTH OF :

	BREAKFAST	LUNCH	DINNER	SNACKS	NOTES
MONDAY					
TUESDAY					
WEDNESDAY					
THURSDAY					
FRIDAY					
SATURDAY					
SUNDAY					

Fitness Workout Planner

Date: Year: Month:

	Activity	Reps
Day 1		
Day 2		
Day 3		
Day 4		
Day 5		
Day 6		
Day 7		

Weekly
PLAN

WEEK: �957

SUNDAY	
MONDAY	
TUESDAY	
WEDNESDAY	
THURSDAY	
FRIDAY	
SATURDAY	

To do

- ☐ ....
- ☐ ....
- ☐ ....
- ☐ ....
- ☐ ....
- ☐ ....
- ☐ ....
- ☐ ....

Tracker

S	M	T	W	T	F	S
☐	☐	☐	☐	☐	☐	☐
☐	☐	☐	☐	☐	☐	☐
☐	☐	☐	☐	☐	☐	☐

Notes

....
....
....
....
....
....
....
....

MY JOURNAL

WEEKLY REVIEW

Date: _____

Week: 1 2 3 4

HOW WAS THE WEEK?

FELT GRATEFUL THIS WEEK FOR:

THIS WEEK'S SMALL WINS

THINGS I HAVE IMPROVED ON:

TASK IN PROGRESS

THIS WEEK'S BAD EXPERIENCE:

WHAT TO NOTE THIS WEEK:

MY JOURNAL

WEEKLY WRITING

Date: ....

Week: 1 2 3 4

HELLO JOURNAL, MY WEEK IS…

MY NOTES

WEEKLY MEAL GOAL

MONTH OF :

	BREAKFAST	LUNCH	DINNER	SNACKS	NOTES
MONDAY					
TUESDAY					
WEDNESDAY					
THURSDAY					
FRIDAY					
SATURDAY					
SUNDAY					

Fitness Workout Planner

Date: Year: Month:

	Activity	Reps
Day 1		
Day 2		
Day 3		
Day 4		
Day 5		
Day 6		
Day 7		

Weekly
PLAN

WEEK:

SUNDAY	
MONDAY	
TUESDAY	
WEDNESDAY	
THURSDAY	
FRIDAY	
SATURDAY	

To do

-
-
-
-
-
-
-
-

Tracker

S	M	T	W	T	F	S
S	M	T	W	T	F	S
S	M	T	W	T	F	S

Notes

MY JOURNAL

WEEKLY REVIEW

HOW WAS THE WEEK?

FELT GRATEFUL THIS WEEK FOR:

THIS WEEK'S SMALL WINS

THINGS I HAVE IMPROVED ON:

TASK IN PROGRESS

THIS WEEK'S BAD EXPERIENCE:

WHAT TO NOTE THIS WEEK:

MY JOURNAL

WEEKLY WRITING

Date: ....

Week: 1 2 3 4

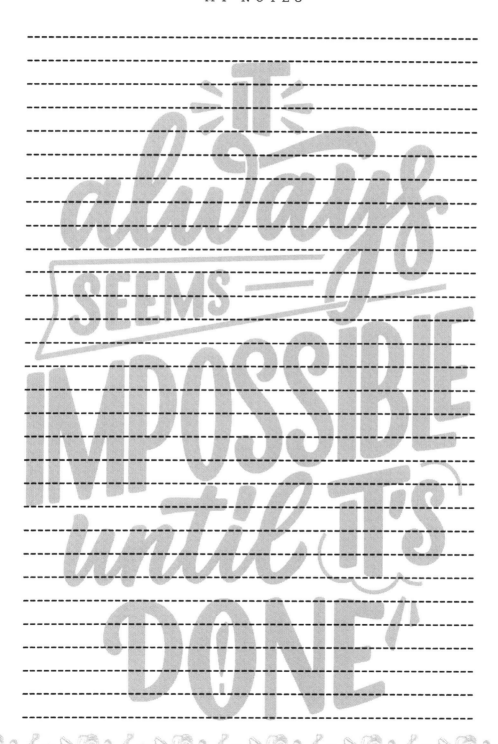

WEEKLY MEAL GOAL

MONTH OF :

	BREAKFAST	LUNCH	DINNER	SNACKS	NOTES
MONDAY					
TUESDAY					
WEDNESDAY					
THURSDAY					
FRIDAY					
SATURDAY					
SUNDAY					

Fitness Workout Planner

Date: Year: Month:

	Activity	Reps
Day 1		
Day 2		
Day 3		
Day 4		
Day 5		
Day 6		
Day 7		

Weekly
PLAN

WEEK: ▓▓▓▓▓▓▓▓▓

SUNDAY

MONDAY

TUESDAY

WEDNESDAY

THURSDAY

FRIDAY

SATURDAY

To do

- ☐ _____
- ☐ _____
- ☐ _____
- ☐ _____
- ☐ _____
- ☐ _____
- ☐ _____
- ☐ _____

Tracker

S	M	T	W	T	F	S
☐	☐	☐	☐	☐	☐	☐

S	M	T	W	T	F	S
☐	☐	☐	☐	☐	☐	☐

S	M	T	W	T	F	S
☐	☐	☐	☐	☐	☐	☐

Notes

MY JOURNAL

WEEKLY REVIEW

Date: ....

Week: 1 2 3 4

HOW WAS THE WEEK?

FELT GRATEFUL THIS WEEK FOR:

THIS WEEK'S SMALL WINS

THINGS I HAVE IMPROVED ON:

TASK IN PROGRESS

THIS WEEK'S BAD EXPERIENCE:

WHAT TO NOTE THIS WEEK:

MY JOURNAL

WEEKLY WRITING

Date: ....

Week: 1 2 3 4

HELLO JOURNAL, MY WEEK IS...

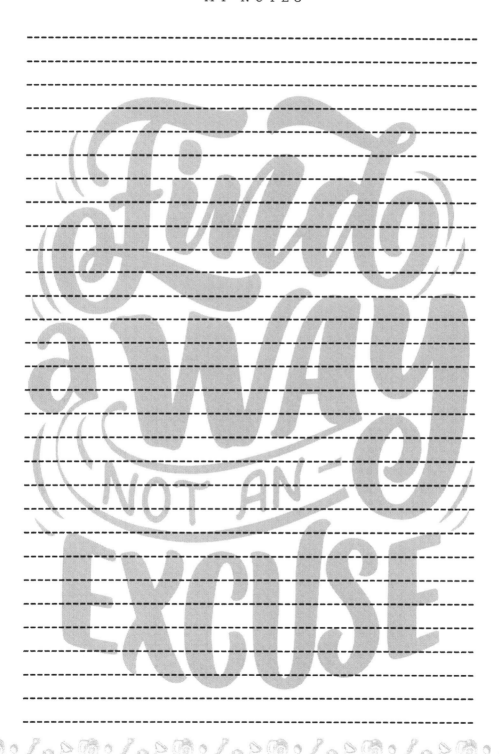

Monthly
PLAN

MONTH:

SUNDAY					
MONDAY					
TUESDAY					
WEDNESDAY					
THURSDAY					
FRIDAY					
SATURDAY					

WEEKLY MEAL GOAL

MONTH OF :

	BREAKFAST	LUNCH	DINNER	SNACKS	NOTES
MONDAY					
TUESDAY					
WEDNESDAY					
THURSDAY					
FRIDAY					
SATURDAY					
SUNDAY					

Fitness Workout Planner

Date: Year: Month:

	Activity	Reps
Day 1		
Day 2		
Day 3		
Day 4		
Day 5		
Day 6		
Day 7		

Weekly
PLAN

WEEK:

SUNDAY

MONDAY

TUESDAY

WEDNESDAY

THURSDAY

FRIDAY

SATURDAY

To do

Tracker

S M T W T F S

S M T W T F S

S M T W T F S

Notes

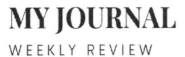

MY JOURNAL

WEEKLY REVIEW

Date: ....

Week: 1 2 3 4

HOW WAS THE WEEK?

FELT GRATEFUL THIS WEEK FOR:

THIS WEEK'S SMALL WINS

THINGS I HAVE IMPROVED ON:

TASK IN PROGRESS

THIS WEEK'S BAD EXPERIENCE:

WHAT TO NOTE THIS WEEK:

MY JOURNAL

WEEKLY WRITING

HELLO JOURNAL, MY WEEK IS...

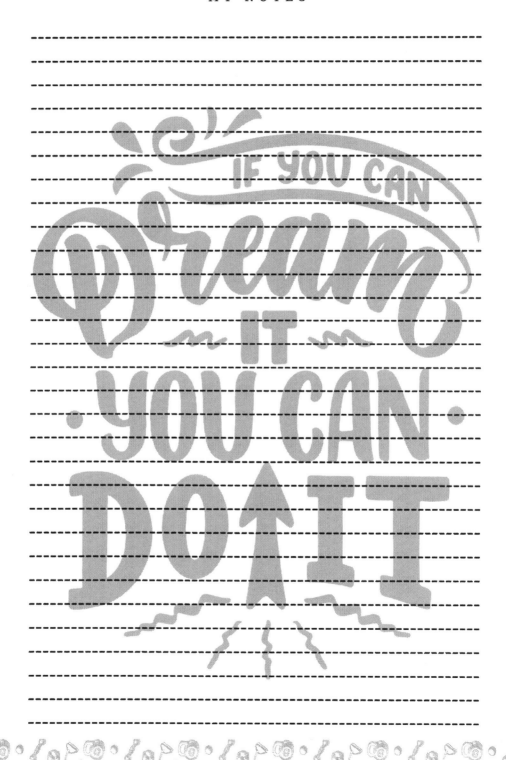

WEEKLY MEAL GOAL

MONTH OF :

	BREAKFAST	LUNCH	DINNER	SNACKS	NOTES
MONDAY					
TUESDAY					
WEDNESDAY					
THURSDAY					
FRIDAY					
SATURDAY					
SUNDAY					

Fitness Workout Planner

Date: Year: Month:

	Activity	Reps
Day 1		
Day 2		
Day 3		
Day 4		
Day 5		
Day 6		
Day 7		

Weekly
PLAN

WEEK:

SUNDAY

MONDAY

TUESDAY

WEDNESDAY

THURSDAY

FRIDAY

SATURDAY

To do

Tracker

S M T W T F S

S M T W T F S

S M T W T F S

Notes

MY JOURNAL

WEEKLY REVIEW

Date: ....

Week: 1 2 3 4

HOW WAS THE WEEK?

FELT GRATEFUL THIS WEEK FOR:

THIS WEEK'S SMALL WINS

THINGS I HAVE IMPROVED ON:

TASK IN PROGRESS

THIS WEEK'S BAD EXPERIENCE:

WHAT TO NOTE THIS WEEK:

MY JOURNAL

WEEKLY WRITING

HELLO JOURNAL, MY WEEK IS...

WEEKLY MEAL GOAL

MONTH OF :

	BREAKFAST	LUNCH	DINNER	SNACKS	NOTES
MONDAY					
TUESDAY					
WEDNESDAY					
THURSDAY					
FRIDAY					
SATURDAY					
SUNDAY					

Fitness Workout Planner

Date: Year: Month:

	Activity	Reps
Day 1		
Day 2		
Day 3		
Day 4		
Day 5		
Day 6		
Day 7		

Weekly

PLAN

WEEK:

SUNDAY

MONDAY

TUESDAY

WEDNESDAY

THURSDAY

FRIDAY

SATURDAY

To do

Tracker

S	M	T	W	T	F	S

S	M	T	W	T	F	S

S	M	T	W	T	F	S

Notes

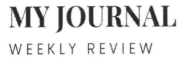

MY JOURNAL

WEEKLY REVIEW

Date: _____

Week: 1 2 3 4

HOW WAS THE WEEK?

FELT GRATEFUL THIS WEEK FOR:

THIS WEEK'S SMALL WINS

THINGS I HAVE IMPROVED ON:

TASK IN PROGRESS

THIS WEEK'S BAD EXPERIENCE:

WHAT TO NOTE THIS WEEK:

MY JOURNAL

WEEKLY WRITING

Date: ....

Week: 1 2 3 4

HELLO JOURNAL, MY WEEK IS...

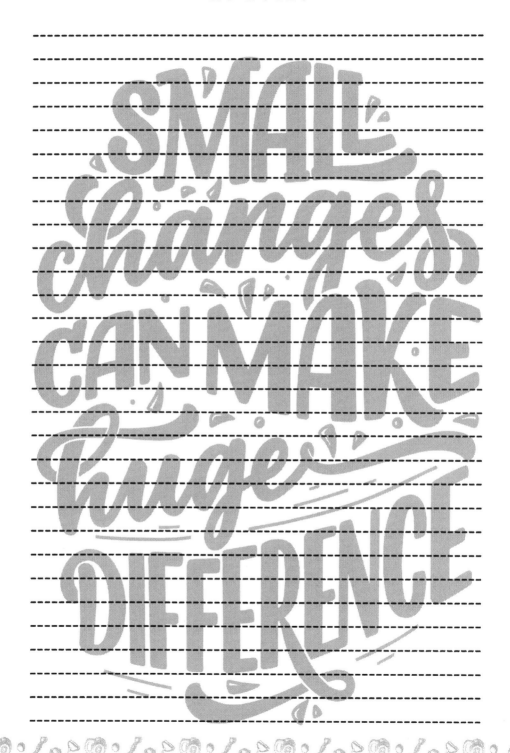

WEEKLY MEAL GOAL

MONTH OF :

	BREAKFAST	LUNCH	DINNER	SNACKS	NOTES
MONDAY					
TUESDAY					
WEDNESDAY					
THURSDAY					
FRIDAY					
SATURDAY					
SUNDAY					

Fitness Workout Planner

Date: Year: Month:

	Activity	Reps
Day 1		
Day 2		
Day 3		
Day 4		
Day 5		
Day 6		
Day 7		

Weekly

PLAN

WEEK: ▮▮▮▮▮▮▮▮▮▮

SUNDAY

MONDAY

TUESDAY

WEDNESDAY

THURSDAY

FRIDAY

SATURDAY

To do

- ▢ ....
- ▢ ....
- ▢ ....
- ▢ ....
- ▢ ....
- ▢ ....
- ▢ ....
- ▢ ....

Tracker

S	M	T	W	T	F	S
▢	▢	▢	▢	▢	▢	▢

S	M	T	W	T	F	S
▢	▢	▢	▢	▢	▢	▢

S	M	T	W	T	F	S
▢	▢	▢	▢	▢	▢	▢

Notes

MY JOURNAL

WEEKLY REVIEW

Date: _____

Week: 1 2 3 4

HOW WAS THE WEEK?

FELT GRATEFUL THIS WEEK FOR:

THIS WEEK'S SMALL WINS

THINGS I HAVE IMPROVED ON:

TASK IN PROGRESS

THIS WEEK'S BAD EXPERIENCE:

WHAT TO NOTE THIS WEEK:

MY JOURNAL

WEEKLY WRITING

Date: ....

Week: 1 2 3 4

HELLO JOURNAL, MY WEEK IS...

Things Take Time

Monthly
PLAN

MONTH:

SUNDAY				
MONDAY				
TUESDAY				
WEDNESDAY				
THURSDAY				
FRIDAY				
SATURDAY				

WEEKLY MEAL GOAL

MONTH OF :

	BREAKFAST	LUNCH	DINNER	SNACKS	NOTES
MONDAY					
TUESDAY					
WEDNESDAY					
THURSDAY					
FRIDAY					
SATURDAY					
SUNDAY					

Fitness Workout Planner

Date: Year: Month:

	Activity	Reps
Day 1		
Day 2		
Day 3		
Day 4		
Day 5		
Day 6		
Day 7		

Weekly
PLAN

SUNDAY	
MONDAY	
TUESDAY	
WEDNESDAY	
THURSDAY	
FRIDAY	
SATURDAY	

To do

Tracker

S M T W T F S

S M T W T F S

S M T W T F S

Notes

MY JOURNAL

WEEKLY REVIEW

HOW WAS THE WEEK?

FELT GRATEFUL THIS WEEK FOR:

THIS WEEK'S SMALL WINS

THINGS I HAVE IMPROVED ON:

TASK IN PROGRESS

THIS WEEK'S BAD EXPERIENCE:

WHAT TO NOTE THIS WEEK:

MY JOURNAL

WEEKLY WRITING

Date: _____

Week: 1 2 3 4

HELLO JOURNAL, MY WEEK IS...

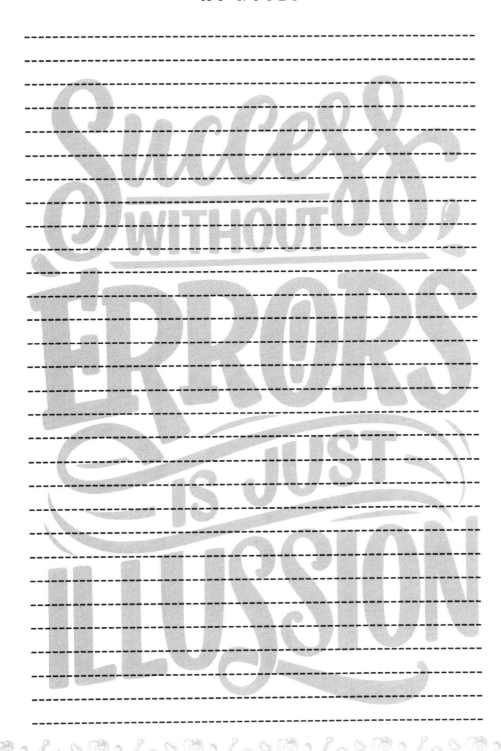

WEEKLY MEAL GOAL

MONTH OF :

	BREAKFAST	LUNCH	DINNER	SNACKS	NOTES
MONDAY					
TUESDAY					
WEDNESDAY					
THURSDAY					
FRIDAY					
SATURDAY					
SUNDAY					

Fitness Workout Planner

Date: Year: Month:

	Activity	Reps
Day 1		
Day 2		
Day 3		
Day 4		
Day 5		
Day 6		
Day 7		

Weekly
PLAN

SUNDAY

MONDAY

TUESDAY

WEDNESDAY

THURSDAY

FRIDAY

SATURDAY

To do

-
-
-
-
-
-
-
-

Tracker

S	M	T	W	T	F	S
S	M	T	W	T	F	S
S	M	T	W	T	F	S

Notes

MY JOURNAL

WEEKLY REVIEW

Date: _____

Week: 1   2   3   4

HOW WAS THE WEEK?

FELT GRATEFUL THIS WEEK FOR:

THIS WEEK'S SMALL WINS

THINGS I HAVE IMPROVED ON:

TASK IN PROGRESS

THIS WEEK'S BAD EXPERIENCE:

WHAT TO NOTE THIS WEEK:

MY JOURNAL

WEEKLY WRITING

Date: ....

Week: 1 2 3 4

HELLO JOURNAL, MY WEEK IS...

WEEKLY MEAL GOAL

MONTH OF :

	BREAKFAST	LUNCH	DINNER	SNACKS	NOTES
MONDAY					
TUESDAY					
WEDNESDAY					
THURSDAY					
FRIDAY					
SATURDAY					
SUNDAY					

Fitness Workout Planner

Date: Year: Month:

	Activity	Reps
Day 1		
Day 2		
Day 3		
Day 4		
Day 5		
Day 6		
Day 7		

Weekly
PLAN

WEEK:

SUNDAY	
MONDAY	
TUESDAY	
WEDNESDAY	
THURSDAY	
FRIDAY	
SATURDAY	

To do

-
-
-
-
-
-
-
-

Tracker

S	M	T	W	T	F	S
S	M	T	W	T	F	S
S	M	T	W	T	F	S

Notes

MY JOURNAL

WEEKLY REVIEW

Date: ....

Week: 1   2   3   4

HOW WAS THE WEEK?	FELT GRATEFUL THIS WEEK FOR:

THIS WEEK'S SMALL WINS	THINGS I HAVE IMPROVED ON:

TASK IN PROGRESS	THIS WEEK'S BAD EXPERIENCE:

WHAT TO NOTE THIS WEEK:

MY JOURNAL

WEEKLY WRITING

Date: ....

Week: 1 2 3 4

HELLO JOURNAL, MY WEEK IS...

WEEKLY MEAL GOAL

MONTH OF :

	BREAKFAST	LUNCH	DINNER	SNACKS	NOTES
MONDAY					
TUESDAY					
WEDNESDAY					
THURSDAY					
FRIDAY					
SATURDAY					
SUNDAY					

Fitness Workout Planner

Date: Year: Month:

	Activity	Reps
Day 1		
Day 2		
Day 3		
Day 4		
Day 5		
Day 6		
Day 7		

Weekly

PLAN

WEEK:

	To do
SUNDAY	☐ _____
	☐ _____
	☐ _____
MONDAY	☐ _____
	☐ _____
	☐ _____
TUESDAY	☐ _____
	☐ _____

Tracker

S M T W T F S

S M T W T F S

S M T W T F S

WEDNESDAY

THURSDAY

Notes

FRIDAY

SATURDAY

MY JOURNAL

WEEKLY REVIEW

Date: ....

Week: 1 2 3 4

HOW WAS THE WEEK?

FELT GRATEFUL THIS WEEK FOR:

THIS WEEK'S SMALL WINS

THINGS I HAVE IMPROVED ON:

TASK IN PROGRESS

THIS WEEK'S BAD EXPERIENCE:

WHAT TO NOTE THIS WEEK:

MY JOURNAL

WEEKLY WRITING

Date: _____

Week: 1   2   3   4

MY NOTES

MY NOTES

MY NOTES

MY NOTES

MY NOTES

MY NOTES

MY NOTES

MY NOTES

MY NOTES

MY NOTES

Made in the USA
Coppell, TX
03 November 2022

85712449R00068